Gluten Free Cake Recipes

A Cookbook for Wheat Free Baking

About the Author

Laura Sommers is **The Recipe Lady!**

She is the #1 Best Selling Author of over 80 recipe books.

She is a loving wife and mother who lives on a small farm in Baltimore County, Maryland and has a passion for all things domestic especially when it comes to saving money. She has a profitable eBay business and is a couponing addict, avid blogger and YouTuber.

Follow her tips and tricks to learn how to make delicious meals on a budget, save money or to learn the latest life hack!

Visit her blog for even more great recipes and to learn which books are FREE for download each week:

http://the-recipe-lady.blogspot.com/

Follow the Recipe Lady on **Pinterest**:

http://pinterest.com/therecipelady1

Visit her Amazon Author Page to see her latest books:

amazon.com/author/laurasommers

© Copyright 2016. Laura Sommers.
All rights reserved.
No part of this book may be reproduced in any form or by any electronic or mechanical means without written permission of the author. All text, illustrations and design are the exclusive property of
Laura Sommers

About the Author ii

Introduction 1

Preventing Contamination 2

Gluten Free Flour Blend 3

Gluten Free Vanilla Cake 4

Gluten Free Strawberry Shortcake 6

Gluten Free Coconut Cake 7

Gluten Free Chocolate Cake 8

Gluten Free Apple Cake...9

Gluten Free Red Velvet Cake 10

Gluten Free Caramel Apple Cake 12

Gluten Free Mexican Wedding Cake 13

Gluten Free Pineapple Upside Down Cake 14

Gluten Free Raspberry Almond Cake 15

Gluten Free Orange Almond Cake...16

Gluten Free Pumpkin Cream Cheese Cake.......................................17

Gluten Free Angel Food Cake 18

Gluten Free White Cake 20

Gluten Free Lemon Cake...22

Gluten Free Marble Cake 24

Gluten Free Rainbow Layer Cake 26

Gluten Free Buttercream Frosting 27

Gluten Free German Chocolate Cake 28

Gluten Free Zucchini Cake...30

Gluten Free Strawberry Cake 32

Gluten Free Gingerbread Cake 33
Gluten Free Carrot Cake 34
Gluten Free Yellow Cake 35
Gluten Free Oatmeal Chocolate Chip Cake 36
Gluten Free Rhubarb Upside Down Cake 37
Gluten Free Blueberry Lemon Pound Cake 38
Gluten Free Coffee Cake 40
About the Author 41
Other books in This Series 42

Introduction

Eating gluten free needn't mean you have to give up your favorite things! You can still enjoy all your favorite cakes but in a gluten free version! No sacrificing of taste.

Get the best gluten free cake recipes in this book!
Discover delicious gluten free cake recipes the whole family will love! Great recipes for those with gluten intolerance, celiac disease, or who are eating a gluten-free diet for other reasons.

Each gluten free cake recipe in this cookbook is easy to prepare with step-by-step instructions. So if you have a wheat allergy or have gluten intolerance, there are many wonderful recipes in this book to give you lots and lots of options to enjoy!

Preventing Contamination

When you have a gluten or wheat allergy or you are just gluten intolerant, you have to be very careful about cross contamination, especially if others in your family don't share your quest for a gluten free life style. Here are some things to be aware of to prevent wheat products from accidentally getting in to your gluten free products.

Keep all you gluten free items in an air tight container.
Wash all surfaces thoroughly before making any gluten free products.
Ideally, have a separate work area or counter that is reserved for gluten free only items.
Have a separate cabinet for anything gluten free and have a strict rule that it is gluten free only!
Lable all gluten free items clearly as Gluten Free.
Have a separate section of the refrigerator or a completely separate refrigerator if possible for all gluten free items.
Have your own container of butter or margarine. A very common culprit of cross contamination is someone buttering their wheat based toast with butter and then sticking the knife back in the butter or scraping the excess off the sides in to the tub of butter.
Have a separate toaster and keep it on a separate counter away from the "gluten toaster." Try to keep both toasters clean but away from each other.

Those are a few tips and tricks to help prevent cross contamination. I hope that they were helpful.

Gluten Free Flour Blend

Ingredients:

2 cups rice flour
2/3 cup potato starch
1/3 cup tapioca flour
1 tsp. xanthan gum

Directions:

Whisk all ingredients together.
Store in an air tight container until ready to use.
Stir before using
Use in the recipes included in this cookbook.

Gluten Free Vanilla Cake

Ingredients:

2 cups all-purpose gluten free flour blend
1 tsp. xanthan gum (omit if your blend already contains it)
1/4 cup + 2 tbsp. cornstarch
1/2 tsp. baking soda
2 tsps. baking powder
1/2 tsp. kosher salt
10 tbsp. unsalted butter, at room temperature
1 1/2 cups granulated sugar
2 tsps. pure vanilla extract
4 egg whites + 1 whole egg, at room temperature
1 1/3 cups buttermilk, at room temperature

Directions:

1. Preheat your oven to 350 degrees F.
2. Grease 2 8-inch round cake pans and line the bottom of each with a round of parchment paper.
3. Set the pans aside.
4. Into a medium-size bowl, sift the flour, xanthan gum, cornstarch, baking soda and baking powder.
5. Add the salt, and whisk to combine well.
6. Set the dry ingredients aside.
7. In the bowl of a stand mixer fitted with the paddle attachment, beat the butter, sugar and vanilla on medium-high speed for at least 3 minutes, stopping at least once to scrape the entire mixture off the sides and bottom of the bowl, or until very light and fluffy.
8. Whisk together the egg whites, egg and buttermilk in a small bowl.
9. Add the dry ingredients and the wet ingredients to the butter and sugar mixture. Start with the dry and alternate dry, wet, dry, wet, dry, wet, dry. Mix in between each addition.
10. The batter will sometimes look a bit curdled.
11. Once all of the ingredients have been added, beat for another minute on medium speed to ensure that everything is combined.
12. Turn over the batter a few times by hand.

13. Divide the batter evenly between the two prepared baking pans and smooth each into an even layer with a spatula.
14. Place the baking pans in the center of the preheated oven and bake for 20 minutes.
15. Rotate the pans, and continue to bake until the cakes are lightly golden brown all over, have begun to pull away from the sides of the pan, about another 10 minutes.
16. Remove the cakes from the oven and allow to cool in the pans for 15 minutes before turning out onto a wire rack and removing the parchment paper liners.
17. Let cool completely before frosting and serving.
18. Serve and enjoy!

Gluten Free Strawberry Shortcake

Ingredients:

2/3 cup brown rice flour
2/3 cup cornstarch
2/3 cup tapioca flour
1 tbsp. baking powder
1/4 tsp. baking soda
1/4 tsp. xanthan gum
1/2 tsp. salt
6 tbsp. vegetable shortening
2/3 cup white sugar
3/4 cup skim milk
4 cups sliced fresh strawberries
2 cups reduced-fat whipped topping

Directions:

1. Preheat an oven to 425 degrees F. (220 degrees C).
2. Whisk the rice flour, cornstarch, tapioca flour, baking powder, baking soda, xanthan gum, and salt together in a bowl.
3. Set aside.
4. Grease a baking sheet, or cover with a sheet of parchment paper.
5. Beat the shortening and sugar with an electric mixer in a large bowl until light and fluffy.
6. Pour in the flour mixture alternately with the milk, mixing until just incorporated.
7. Drop onto the prepared baking sheet into 8 equal portions.
8. Bake until golden brown on the bottoms, 10 to 12 minutes.
9. Remove, and cool on a wire rack to room temperature.
10. Once cool, slice each shortcake in half, and place each bottom half onto a dessert plate.
11. Evenly divide the sliced strawberries onto each shortcake, and dollop with the whipped topping.
12. Place the shortcake tops on to serve.
13. Serve and enjoy!

Gluten Free Coconut Cake

Ingredients:

2 cups gluten-free flour
1 1/2 cups white sugar
1 cup flaked coconut
1/2 cup chopped walnuts
1 tbsp. baking powder
1 tsp. baking soda
1 tsp. xanthan gum
1 tsp. salt 1 cup coconut milk
1 cup vegetable oil 4 eggs
1 tsp. vanilla extract

Directions:

1. Preheat oven to 350 degrees F (175 degrees C).
2. Grease and flour a 9x13-inch baking dish.
3. Whisk flour, sugar, coconut, walnuts, baking powder, baking soda, xanthan gum, and salt together in a bowl.
4. Add coconut milk, vegetable oil, eggs, and vanilla extract; mix until batter is smooth.
5. Spread batter into the prepared baking dish.
6. Bake in the preheated oven until a toothpick inserted in the center comes out clean, about 45 minutes.
7. Serve and enjoy!

Gluten Free Chocolate Cake

Ingredients:

Cooking spray
3 cups gluten-free all-purpose baking flour
2 cups white sugar
1/3 cup cocoa powder
2 1/4 tsps. baking powder
1 1/2 tsps. baking soda
1 1/2 tsps. xanthan gum
1 1/2 cups mayonnaise
1 1/2 cups hot water
1 1/2 tsps. vanilla extract

Directions:

1. Preheat oven to 350 degrees F (175 degrees C).
2. Spray two 9-inch cake pans with cooking spray.
3. Combine flour, sugar, cocoa powder, baking powder, baking soda, and xanthan gum in a bowl.
4. Stir in mayonnaise until well mixed.
5. Gradually pour in hot water and vanilla extract; stir until smooth.
6. Spoon batter into the prepared cake pans.
7. Bake in the preheated oven until a toothpick inserted in the center of the cake comes out clean and the cake slightly pulls away from the sides of the pan, about 30 minutes.
8. Cool in the pans for 10 minutes before removing to cool completely on a wire rack.
9. Serve and enjoy!

Gluten Free Apple Cake

Ingredients:

3/4 cup sorghum flour
3/4 cup almond flour
1/4 cup rice flour
1/4 cup tapioca flour
1 tbsp. xanthan gum
1 tsp. ground cinnamon
1 tsp. baking soda
1/2 tsp. baking powder
1/2 tsp. salt
1 3/4 cups white sugar
1 cup vegetable oil
3 eggs
4 small Golden Delicious apples, peeled, cored, and chopped
1/2 cup coarsely chopped walnuts

Directions:

1. Preheat oven to 350 degrees F (175 degrees C).
2. Grease a 9x13-inch pan; lightly flour with gluten-free flour.
3. Whisk sorghum flour, almond flour, rice flour, tapioca flour, xanthan gum, cinnamon, baking soda, baking powder, and salt together in a bowl.
4. Whisk sugar, vegetable oil, and eggs together in a separate bowl.
5. Stir into flour mixture until incorporated and batter is thoroughly combined.
6. Fold in apples and walnuts.
7. Pour and press batter into the prepared pan.
8. Bake in the preheated oven until a knife inserted into the middle of the cake comes out clean, about 1 hour.
9. Serve and enjoy!

Gluten Free Red Velvet Cake

Ingredients:

3/4 cup brown rice flour
1/4 cup coconut flour
3/4 cup sorghum flour
3/4 cup tapioca starch
1 tsp. baking soda
1 tsp. xanthan gum
1/4 tsp. salt
1/4 cup unsweetened cocoa powder, divided
1 cup canola oil
1 1/2 cups white sugar
2 eggs at room temperature
3/4 cup unsweetened applesauce
1 cup buttermilk
1 oz. red food coloring
1 tsp. vanilla extract

Directions:

1. Preheat oven to 350 degrees F. (175 degrees C).
2. Grease and flour 2 9" round cake pans with gluten-free flour.
3. In a bowl, whisk together the brown rice flour, coconut flour, sorghum flour, tapioca starch, baking soda, xanthan gum, salt, and 3 tbsp. of cocoa powder.
4. In a large mixing bowl, beat canola oil and sugar until thoroughly combined, and beat the eggs in one at a time until fully incorporated.
5. Stir in the applesauce.
6. Beat the flour mixture into the wet ingredients, alternating with buttermilk, in several additions, beginning and ending with flour mixture.
7. Mix the remaining 1 tbsp. of cocoa powder with the red food coloring and vanilla extract to make a paste.
8. Gently stir into the batter.
9. Pour the batter into the prepared cake pans.
10. Bake in the preheated oven until a toothpick inserted into the center of a cake comes out clean, about 25 minutes.

11. Allow the cakes to cool completely before frosting.
12. Serve and enjoy!

Gluten Free Caramel Apple Cake

Ingredients:

1 1/2 cups vanilla yogurt 1 cup white sugar 1 cup brown sugar 3 eggs 2 tsps. vanilla extract 3 cups gluten-free all-purpose baking flour 3 tbsp. ground flax seed 1 tsp. ground cinnamon 1 tsp. salt 1/8 tsp. ground cloves 1/8 tsp. ground nutmeg 4 apples, shredded
Caramel Sauce: 1/2 cup butter 1/2 cup brown sugar
2 tsps. milk

Directions:

1. Preheat oven to 325 degrees F (165 degrees C). Grease a fluted tube pan (such as Bundt(R)).
2. Beat yogurt, white sugar, 1 cup brown sugar, eggs, and vanilla extract together in a bowl using an electric mixer until smooth.
3. Combine flour, flax seed, cinnamon, salt, cloves, and nutmeg together in a separate bowl. Stir yogurt mixture into flour mixture just until batter is combined; fold in apples. Pour batter into prepared pan.
4. Bake in the preheated oven until a toothpick inserted in the center of the cake comes out clean, 70 to 75 minutes. Turn cake onto a serving plate.
5. Melt butter, 1/2 cup brown sugar, and milk together in a saucepan over medium heat until sugar is dissolved, 2 to 3 minutes. Remove saucepan from heat and cool until sauce is thickened, about 10 minutes. Pour sauce over cake.
6. Serve and enjoy!

Gluten Free Mexican Wedding Cake

Ingredients:

1/2 cup butter
1 tsp. gluten free vanilla extract
1 cup confectioners' sugar
1/2 cup white rice flour
1/4 cup cornstarch
1/4 cup tapioca flour
1/4 tsp. unflavored gelatin (optional)
1 cup chopped hazelnuts
1 cup chopped walnuts or hazelnuts
Confectioners' sugar for dusting

Directions:

1. Preheat the oven to 350 degrees F (175 degrees C).
2. In a medium bowl, mix together the butter and vanilla until well blended. Sift together the confectioners' sugar, rice flour, cornstarch, tapioca starch and gelatin. Stir into the butter mixture until all of the dry ingredients have been absorbed. Mix in the ground hazelnuts and chopped hazelnuts. Form teaspoonfuls of dough into balls, and shape into crescents. Place cookies at least 2 inches apart onto ungreased cookie sheets.
3. Bake for 8 to 10 minutes in the preheated oven, until golden brown. For crispier cookies, reduce heat to 325 degrees F (165 degrees C), and bake slightly longer. When cookies have cooled completely, dust with additional confectioners' sugar.
4. Serve and enjoy!

Gluten Free Pineapple Upside Down Cake

Ingredients:

1 1/2 cups brown sugar
1/2 cup butter 1/4 cup sweet vermouth
1/2 (14 oz.) can pitted dark sweet cherries, drained and halved
1 (20 oz.) can crushed pineapple, drained well and juice reserved
Cake:
3 large eggs
1/2 cup melted butter
1/2 cup pineapple juice
2 tsps. vanilla extract
1 tsp. ground star anise
1 (19 oz.) package gluten-free vanilla cake mix

Directions:

1. Preheat oven to 325 degrees F (165 degrees C).
2. Combine brown sugar, 1/2 cup butter, and sweet vermouth in a saucepan over low heat; cook and stir until sugar is dissolved, about 5 minutes.
3. Arrange cherries and spoon pineapple into the bottom of a 9x13-inch baking dish. Pour brown sugar mixture over fruit.
4. Beat eggs in a bowl using an electric mixer on medium-low speed until smooth. Add 1/2 cup melted butter, pineapple juice, vanilla extract, and star anise to eggs; beat on medium-low speed until well combined, about 1 minute. Gradually add cake mix, about 1/2 cup at a time, to egg mixture, scraping sides of bowl with a spatula until batter is smooth and fluffy. Pour batter over fruit mixture until evenly spread in dish.
5. Bake in the preheated oven until cake is golden brown and completely set in the middle, about 1 hour. Cool cake for 15 minutes in the dish. Run a knife along the edge of the cake to loosen. Place a platter over the cake and flip cake onto platter.
6. Serve and enjoy!

Gluten Free Raspberry Almond Cake

Ingredients:

1 cup blanched almond flour 2 tbsp. coconut flour 1/2 tsp. baking soda 1/4 tsp. salt 3 eggs 1/4 cup butter, melted 1/4 cup honey 1 tbsp. vanilla extract 1/2 cup raspberry jam 1/2 cup slivered almonds Almond Icing: 1/2 cup confectioners' sugar 1 tbsp. milk
1/2 tsp. almond extract

Directions:

1. Preheat oven to 350 degrees F (175 degrees C).
2. Grease a 12x8-inch baking dish.
3. Stir almond flour, coconut flour, baking soda, and salt together in a bowl. Beat eggs, melted butter, honey, and vanilla extract together in a large bowl until smooth; add flour mixture and mix into a dough ball.
4. Split 2/3 of the dough from the ball; spread into the bottom of the prepared baking dish to cover completely. Spoon raspberry jam atop the dough and spread to cover. Break remaining dough into small pieces and dot jam with the dough. Sprinkle almonds over the dough and jam.
5. Bake in the preheated oven until a toothpick inserted into the center comes out clean, about 25 minutes. Cool cake slightly, 10 to 15 minutes.
6. Beat confectioners' sugar, milk, and almond extract together in a small bowl; drizzle over cooled cake.
7. Serve and enjoy!

Gluten Free Orange Almond Cake

Ingredients:

3 eggs, separated 2/3 cup white sugar 1/4 cup rice flour 1 tsp. ground cinnamon 1/2 cup orange juice 1 1/2 cups finely ground almonds (almond meal) 2 tbsp. heavy cream 2 cups white sugar 1 cup orange juice 1 tbsp. grated orange zest
1/2 cup butter 4 egg whites

Directions:

1. Preheat the oven to 325 degrees F (165 degrees C). Grease a 10 inch springform pan with cooking spray, and dust with rice flour.
2. In a large bowl, whip egg yolks with 2/3 cup of sugar until thick and pale using an electric mixer. This will take about 5 minutes. Stir in the rice flour and orange juice, then fold in the almond meal and cinnamon.
3. In a separate glass or metal bowl, whip 3 egg whites until they can hold a stiff peak. Fold into the almond mixture until well blended. Pour into the prepared pan, and spread evenly.
4. Bake for 35 to 40 minutes in the preheated oven, until a toothpick inserted into the center comes out clean. Cool in the pan on a wire rack. Run a knife around the outer edge of the cake to help remove it from the pan.
5. To make the orange sauce, cream together the butter and 2 cups of white sugar in a medium bowl. Stir in the cream, and place the dish over a pan of barely simmering water. Stir in orange juice and zest. Whip 4 egg whites in a separate bowl until soft peaks form. Fold into the orange sauce. Spoon over the cake and serve immediately.
6. Serve and enjoy!

Gluten Free Pumpkin Cream Cheese Cake

Ingredients:

Cooking spray
1 (8 oz.) package cream cheese, softened
3/4 cup white sugar
1 tbsp. cornstarch
2 cups gluten-free flour blend
1 (15 oz.) can pumpkin puree
1 1/2 cups white sugar
3 eggs
3/4 cup milk
1/2 cup melted butter
1 tbsp. baking powder
1 tbsp. ground cinnamon
1/2 tsp. salt

Directions:

1. Preheat oven to 350 degrees F (175 degrees C).
2. Prepare 2 loaf pans with cooking spray.
3. Beat cream cheese, 3/4 cup sugar, and cornstarch together in a small bowl until creamy and smooth.
4. Beat flour blend, pumpkin puree, 1 1/2 cups sugar, eggs, milk, butter, baking powder, cinnamon, and salt together in a large mixing bowl with an electric hand mixer set to Low until you have a thick batter.
5. Pour about 1/4 of the batter into the bottom of each prepared loaf pan. Spread 1/2 the cream cheese filling over each batter portion. Divide remaining batter between the two pans and spread into an even layer.
6. Bake in the preheated oven until a toothpick inserted into the center of the cake, not the filling, comes out clean, about 1 hour.
7. Serve and enjoy!

Gluten Free Angel Food Cake

Ingredients:

3/4 cup gluten-free multi-purpose flour
3/4 cup superfine sugar
1/4 cup cornstarch
1 1/2 cups egg whites (10 to 11 large eggs, separated)
1/4 teaspoon salt
1 ½ teaspoons cream of tartar
2 teaspoons vanilla extract
1/4 teaspoon almond extract, optional
3/4 cup + 2 tablespoons superfine sugar

Directions:

1. Preheat the oven to 350 degrees F. and place the oven rack in its lowest position.
2. Whisk together and then sift the flour, cornstarch, and 3/4 cup sugar.
3. Set aside.
4. In a large mixing bowl, beat together the egg whites, salt, and cream of tartar until foamy.
5. Add the flavorings.
6. Gradually increase the speed of the mixer and continue beating until the egg whites have increased in volume, and thickened.
7. Gradually beat in the 3/4 cup + 2 tablespoons sugar, a bit at a time, until the meringue holds soft peaks.
8. Gently fold in the sifted flour/sugar blend ¼ cup at a time, just until incorporated.
9. Spoon the batter into an ungreased 10" round angel food pan.
10. Gently tap the pan on the counter to settle the batter and remove any large air bubbles.
11. Bake the cake until it's a deep golden brown, and the top springs back when pressed lightly, about 45 minutes.
12. Remove the cake from the oven and invert the pan onto the neck of a heatproof bottle or funnel, to suspend the cake upside down as it sets and cools, about 2 hours.
13. Remove the cake from the pan by running a thin spatula or knife around the edges of the pan, and turning the cake out onto a plate.

14. Cut the cake with a serrated knife or angel food cake comb. If it's difficult to cut, wet the knife and wipe it clean between slices.
15. Serve with whipped cream and fruit.
16. Serve and enjoy!

Gluten Free White Cake

Cake Ingredients:

1/4 cup coconut flour
2 3/4 cup all-purpose gluten free flour
1 2/3 cup granulated sugar
1 tbsp. GF Baking Powder
3/4 tsp. salt
3/4 cup salted butter, softened
1/2 cup vegetable oil
8 egg whites
1 1/4 cups milk
2 tsps. gluten free vanilla

Pink Buttercream Frosting Ingredients:

4 cups powdered sugar
5 tbsp. milk or half and half
1 tsp. vanilla
1 cup slightly softened butter
Pink Food Coloring (optional)

Cake Directions:

1. Preheat oven to 350 degrees F and grease and flour three 8 inch cake pans or two 9 inch pans, one 9x13 inch pan or a couple dozen cupcakes.
2. Mix the flours, sugar, baking powder, and salt on low speed for a minute to fluff them up.
3. Add the butter and oil and continue mixing for another minute until incorporated.
4. Add the egg whites one at a time, beating well after each addition.
5. Add the milk and vanilla a little at a time and then beat on high speed for two minutes. The batter should be thick and fluffy.
6. Pour the batter into the prepared pans.
7. Bake for about 20 minutes or until a toothpick comes out clean.
8. Cool completely before frosting.

Pink Buttercream Frosting Directions:

1. Combine the sugar, milk, and vanilla.
2. Beat until smooth.
3. Cut the butter into chunks and beat in a handful at a time.
4. Continue beating at high speed for at least five minutes or until all the butter is incorporated and the frosting is fluffy.
5. Add the food coloring until desired color is reached.
6. Use to frost the cake.
7. Serve and enjoy!

Gluten Free Lemon Cake

Ingredients:

4 eggs
2 cups of sugar
1 cup of skim milk
1 cup of olive oil
1 tbsp. of vanilla extract
1/4 cup of lemon juice
2 1/2 cups of gluten-free flour
1 tbsp. of baking powder
1/2 tsp. salt
For the lemon butter icing:
1 cup sweet cream salted butter
3 1/2 cups of confectioners' sugar
1/2 cup of lemon juice
Lemon curd

Directions:

1. Preheat oven to 350 degrees F.
2. Whisk the eggs until well beaten.
3. Mix in the sugar.
4. Add the milk, oil, vanilla extract and lemon juice and mix well.
5. Add the dry ingredients next and mix well. The cake batter will be runny.
6. Spray two 9-inch round cake pans with cooking spray.
7. Pour cake batter in to cake pans.
8. Bake for 30-35 minutes or until golden brown and done in the center when a wooden toothpick inserted into the cake comes out clean.
9. Let the cake cool completely before removing it from the cake pans.
10. At this point you can start on the lemon butter frosting for the cake.
11. In a microwave safe bowl, soften the butter until it is not quite melted.
12. Using a spatula, mix in the confectioners' sugar 1/2 a cup at a time.
13. When about 1 cup of the sugar has been mixed in, add in the lemon juice.
14. Continue to add in the sugar until gone and the icing is thick.

15. Remove the cake from the oven when done and allow to cool completely.
16. Run a knife around the edges of the cake pans to loosen the cake. Gently tap and shake the cake to remove from the pan.
17. Place one of the cakes top side down on a plate or cake stand.
18. Spread a thick layer of lemon curd on top of the first cake layer.
19. Place the second cake on top of the first, this time with the top side up.
20. Scoop a large bit of the lemon butter icing on the top of the cake and then smooth over the sides and top.
21. Serve and enjoy!

Gluten Free Marble Cake

Ingredients:

8 tbsps. unsalted butter, at room temperature
1 cup sugar
3 eggs at room temperature, beaten
2 tsps. pure vanilla extract
2 cups gluten free flour blend
1/2 tsp. xanthan gum
1 tsp. baking powder
1/2 tsp. baking soda
1/2 tsp. kosher salt
2/3 cup milk, at room temperature
1/4 cup natural cocoa powder
2 tbsps. warm water

Directions:

1. Preheat your oven to 325 degrees F.
2. Grease a standard 9-inch x 5-inch (or slightly smaller) loaf pan, and set it aside.
3. In the bowl of a stand mixer fitted with the paddle attachment (or a large bowl with a handheld mixer), cream the butter until light and fluffy. Add the sugar, eggs, and vanilla, mixing well after each addition. In a separate medium-size bowl, whisk together the flour blend, xanthan gum, baking powder, baking soda and salt. Add the flour mixture in 3 parts to the butter mixture, alternating with the milk, mixing until just combined after each addition until all of the flour mixture and milk have been added. The batter should be light and smooth. Scrape half of the batter into a separate, medium-size bowl and set it aside.
4. In a small bowl, place the cocoa powder and warm water and mix together until smooth.
5. Scrape the cocoa mixture into the mixing bowl and mix with the remaining half of the vanilla batter until just combined.
6. Marble the separate batters together in the prepared pan in the following manner:

7. Using ice cream scoops, begin by placing one portion of about 2 tablespoons of vanilla batter to the bottom center of the loaf pan.
8. Shake the pan from side to side gently to spread the batter a bit.
9. Place an equal portion of the chocolate batter in the center of the vanilla batter, and again shake the pan from side to side gently.
10. Place a second portion of vanilla batter in the center of the chocolate batter, shake the pan again gently, and repeat with the chocolate batter, alternating until all the batter is in the pan.
11. Place the pan in the center of the preheated oven and bake until a toothpick inserted in the center comes out clean (about 45 minutes).
12. Remove from the oven and allow the cake, still in the pan, to cool on a wire rack for at least 20 minutes.
13. Carefully remove the cake from the pan, and place it on the wire rack to cool completely.
14. Serve and enjoy!

Gluten Free Rainbow Layer Cake

Ingredients:

2 cups granulated sugar
1 cup vegetable oil
4 eggs
2 tsps. vanilla extract
3 3/4 cups gluten-free flour blend
1 tsp. xanthan gum (omit if your blend already has it)
3/4 tsp. baking soda
1/2 tsp. salt
1 1/2 cups buttermilk
Food coloring (purple, blue, green, yellow, orange, red)
Buttercream frosting (see recipe)

Directions:

1. Preheat the oven to 350 degrees F.
2. Lightly grease 6 9" round baking pans and line the bottom with a circle of parchment paper. (bake in batches if needed)
3. In a stand mixer, beat the sugar and oil until creamy.
4. Add the eggs one at a time.
5. Add the vanilla and beat until light and fluffy.
6. In a separate bowl whisk together the gluten-free flour, xanthan gum, baking soda, and salt.
7. Add the flour mixture to the sugar mixture in 3 additions, alternating with the buttermilk, beginning and ending with the flour mixture.
8. Mix until the batter is smooth.
9. Divide the batter evenly between 6 bowls and color each bowl of batter the desired color using the food coloring.
10. Pour the batter into the prepared pans and bake 2 at a time for about 15-17 minutes or until a toothpick comes out clean.
11. Spread about 1½ cups of frosting between each layer and frost the outside with the remaining frosting.
12. Lay the layers in the following order as you frost: purple, blue, green, yellow, orange and red.
13. Serve and enjoy!

Gluten Free Buttercream Frosting

Ingredients:

4 cups powdered sugar
5 tbsp. milk or half and half
1 tsp. vanilla
1 cup slightly softened butter

Directions:

Combine the sugar, milk, and vanilla.
Beat until smooth.
Cut the butter into chunks and beat in a handful at a time.
Continue beating at high speed for at least five minutes or until all the butter is incorporated and the frosting is fluffy.
Use to frost the cake.
Serve and enjoy!

Gluten Free German Chocolate Cake

Batter Ingredients:

4 oz. sweet baking German chocolate
1/2 cup boiling water
1 cup granulate sugar
1/4 cup oil (any oil you like to use in baking will work)
1/2 cup unsweetened applesauce
2 eggs
2 cups gum free gluten free flour blend
1 tsp. baking soda
½ tsp. salt
1/2 cup buttermilk
2 tsps. pure vanilla extract

Filling Ingredients:

3/4 cup granulated sugar
1 cup milk
1/4 cup butter
2 eggs, beaten
1 tsp. pure vanilla extract
1/2 to 1 cup unsweetened shredded dried coconut
1/2 to 3/4 cup toasted pecans

Directions:

1. Preheat oven to 350 degrees F.
2. Grease two 8 or 9-inch round cake pans.
3. Place chocolate in a small mixing bowl and pour hot water over.
4. Let stand while you begin mixing other cake ingredients.
5. In a stand mixer, combine sugar, oil, applesauce and eggs; mix on low to blend.
6. In a separate bowl, whisk flour, baking soda and salt together.
7. Add dry ingredients to mixing bowl with liquid ingredients.
8. Blend on low at first, then on medium speed until mixture is relatively smooth.

9. Stop mixer and stir the chocolate you poured hot water over. The chocolate will be melted.
10. Add chocolate and water mixture to mixing bowl and blend on low speed until batter is smooth, about 2 – 3 minutes.
11. Add buttermilk and vanilla to the batter and mix on low to blend fully, about 2 more minutes.
12. Divide batter evenly between the two pans and bake about 25 minutes, or until tops of layers appear dry and spring back when gently touched.
13. When layers are done, remove from oven and cool in pan while you prepare the filling.

Filling Directions:

1. Combine sugar, milk, butter and eggs in a medium saucepan.
2. Whisk to blend.
3. Place the saucepan over medium heat and cook and stir until the mixture comes to a gentle boil. If you do not stir, the eggs will curdle.
4. When the mixture begins to boil, and you're still whisking to prevent curdling, you will notice the mixture thickens slightly.
5. Remove the filling from the heat.
6. Add the remaining ingredients and stir.
7. Cool filling to almost room temperature before assembling cake.
8. Remove your cake layers from pans when they are cool enough to handle.
9. Place one layer on a serving plate, top with about 1/4 of the filling Repeat until all layers are used.
10. Top cake with remaining filling.
11. Frost sides if desired.
12. Serve and enjoy!

Gluten Free Zucchini Cake

Ingredients:

1 1/2 cups grated zucchini
1 tsp. vanilla
1 cup raw or organic cane sugar
1 tsp. baking powder
1 tsp. baking soda
1/4 cup olive oil
1/4 cup unsweetened applesauce
2 eggs
1/2 tsp. cinnamon
1 1/2 cups gluten free flour blend
3/4 cup almond meal
1/4 cup gluten free oats
1 pinch salt

Cream Cheese Frosting Ingredients:

4 tbsp. butter, softened
2- 2 1/2 cups powdered sugar
4 oz. softened cream cheese, softened
1/4 tsp. pure vanilla extract

Cake Directions:

1. Preheat oven to 300 degrees F.
2. Grease and flour an 8x8 pan with butter or cooking spray and gluten free flour blend.
3. In a large mixing bowl, whisk together sugar, oil, applesauce, eggs, and zucchini.
4. Add vanilla, baking soda, baking powder and cinnamon.
5. Add almond meal, gluten free flour blend, and gluten free oats and whisk again to combine.
6. Pour batter into your pan and bake for 45 minutes to 1 hour, or when a toothpick inserted comes out clean and the edges are golden brown.
7. Cool completely before frosting.

Frosting Directions:

8. In a bowl, beat the dairy-free butter and cream cheese together.
9. Add vanilla and beat again.
10. Add powdered sugar 1/2 cup at a time until you reach desired consistency and sweetness.
11. Frost the cake once it is cooled.
12. Serve and enjoy!

Gluten Free Strawberry Cake

Ingredients:

3 sticks of butter, softened but not melted
2 3/4 cups granulated white sugar
5 eggs
3 cups gluten free flour blend
1/2 tsp salt
2/3 tsp baking powder
1 tsp. xanthan gum
1 cup milk
1 tsp. almond extract

Directions:

1. Preheat oven to 350 degrees F.
2. Butter and flour a tube or bundt pan.
3. With a mixer, cream butter and sugar together.
4. Add eggs, 1 at a time, beating after each addition.
5. Stir dry ingredients together in a bowl and add to mixer alternately with milk, starting with the flour and ending with the flour.
6. Mix in almond extract.
7. Pour into prepared tube pan and bake for 1 to 1 1/2 hours, until a toothpick inserted in the center of the cake comes out clean.
8. Occasionally peek at the cake though. If they top starts to get really brown, you will need to lay a piece of foil loosely over it so that it can keep cooking internally without burning the top.
9. When it is done, remove it from the oven and let it sit in the pan for 10 minutes before inverting it onto a plate. If you do it sooner, your cake might fall slightly.
10. Serve and enjoy!

Gluten Free Gingerbread Cake

Ingredients:

2 tbsp. ground flax seeds
6 tbsp. warm water
5/6 cup millet flour
5/6 cup teff flour
1/3 cup potato starch (not flour)
1 tsp. gluten-free baking powder
1 tsp. baking soda
2 tsps. ground ginger
1 tsp. ground cinnamon
1/4 tsp. ground cloves
1/4 tsp. salt
2/3 cup coconut palm sugar
1/2 cup unsulfured molasses
1/3 cup coconut oil
1 cup unsweetened applesauce

Directions:

1. Preheat oven to 350 degrees F.
2. Grease an 8x8-inch pan or line it with parchment paper.
3. In a small bowl, stir together the flax and warm water until the mixture is thick and creamy.
4. Set aside for at least 10 minutes.
5. Sift the dry ingredients (except the coconut palm sugar) into a large mixing bowl.
6. In another mixing bowl, combine the coconut palm sugar, molasses, coconut oil, applesauce, and flax mixture; whisk until well blended. Add to the dry ingredients and stir to blend.
7. Pour the batter into the prepared pan. Bake until set in the middle and a tester comes out clean, about 35 minutes.
8. Cool in pan on rack until cake is cool enough to handle, then turn out.
9. Serve and enjoy!

Gluten Free Carrot Cake

Ingredients:

1 1/2 cups white rice flour
3/4 cup tapioca flour
1 tsp. salt
1 tsp. baking soda
3 tsps. baking powder
1 tsp. xanthan gum
4 eggs
1 1/4 cups white sugar
2/3 cup mayonnaise
1 cup milk
2 tsps. gluten free vanilla extract

Directions:

1. Preheat oven to 350 degrees F (175 degrees C).
2. Grease and rice flour two 8 or 9 inch round cake pans.
3. Mix the white rice flour, tapioca flour, salt, baking soda, baking powder and xanthan gum together and set aside.
4. Mix the eggs, sugar, and mayonnaise until fluffy.
5. Add the flour mixture, milk and vanilla and mix well.
6. Spread batter into the prepared pans.
7. Bake at 350 degrees F (175 degrees C) for 25 minutes.
8. Cakes are done when they spring back when lightly touched or when a toothpick inserted near the center comes out clean.
9. Let cool completely then frost, if desired.
10. Serve and enjoy!

Gluten Free Yellow Cake

Ingredients:

1 1/2 cups white rice flour
3/4 cup tapioca flour
1 tsp. salt 1 tsp. baking soda
3 tsps. baking powder
1 tsp. xanthan gum 4 eggs
1 1/4 cups white sugar
2/3 cup mayonnaise
1 cup milk
2 tsps. gluten free vanilla extract

Directions:

1. Preheat oven to 350 degrees F (175 degrees C).
2. Grease and rice flour two 8 or 9 inch round cake pans.
3. Mix the white rice flour, tapioca flour, salt, baking soda, baking powder and xanthan gum together and set aside.
4. Mix the eggs, sugar, and mayonnaise until fluffy.
5. Add the flour mixture, milk and vanilla and mix well.
6. Spread batter into the prepared pans.
7. Bake at 350 degrees F (175 degrees C) for 25 minutes.
8. Cakes are done when they spring back when lightly touched or when a toothpick inserted near the center comes out clean.
9. Let cool completely then frost, if desired.
10. Serve and enjoy!

Gluten Free Oatmeal Chocolate Chip Cake

Ingredients:

1 cup GF rolled oats
6 Tbsp. oil/butter
2 1/4 cups hot water
½-2/3 cup honey
¼ cup ground flax
1 cup brown rice flour
3/4 cup GF oat flour
1 Tbsp. cocoa powder
1 tsp. baking soda
1/2 tsp. sea salt
1 1/2 cup chocolate chips*
3/4 cup chopped walnuts

Directions:

1. Pour hot water over rolled oats and oil/butter in a large bowl.
2. Let set for at least 10 minutes before whisking in the honey and ground flax.
3. Mix the dry ingredients together, and then combine with the wet.
4. Gently fold in about half of the chocolate chips.
5. Pour into a rectangular cake pan.
6. Sprinkle the rest of the chocolate chips plus the chopped walnuts on top.
7. Bake at 35o degrees for 35-40 minutes.
8. Serve and enjoy!

Gluten Free Rhubarb Upside Down Cake

Ingredietns:

1/2 cup butter
1 cup white sugar
3 stalks rhubarb, cut into 1-inch pieces
2 cups gluten-free flour blend
2 tsps. baking soda
1/2 tsp. salt
1 cup yogurt
1/2 cup coconut oil, melted
1 egg
1 tsp. vanilla extract

Directions:

1. Preheat oven to 350 degrees F (175 degrees C).
2. Melt butter in a large cast iron skillet or Dutch oven over medium-low heat.
3. Add sugar and rhubarb; cook until rhubarb is soft, 5 to 8 minutes. Remove from heat.
4. Mix gluten-free flour, baking soda, and salt together in a large bowl.
5. Add yogurt, coconut oil, egg, and vanilla extract; stir thoroughly until batter is combined.
6. Drop cake batter over rhubarb mixture in the skillet.
7. Spread it out gently until mostly smooth.
8. Bake in the preheated oven until top is golden and a toothpick inserted into the center comes out clean, about 25 minutes.
9. Run a knife around the edges, place a plate on top and carefully invert cake onto the plate.
10. Serve and enjoy!

Gluten Free Blueberry Lemon Pound Cake

Cake Ingredients:

2 cups sugar
1 cup butter or margarine, melted
4 eggs
4 tsps. gluten-free vanilla
3 cups Gluten-Free Flour Blend
2 tsps. gluten-free baking powder
1 cup milk
1 tbsp. lemon zest
1/4 cup of freshly squeezed lemon juice
2 cups blueberries
Glaze
1/2 cup sifted powdered sugar
4 tsps. lemon juice

Cake Directions:

1. Heat oven to 350 degrees F.
2. Grease 12-cup Bundt or 10-inch tube pan.
3. Sprinkle with gluten-free flour blend.
4. Set aside.
5. Combine sugar and melted butter in large bowl. Beat at medium speed, scraping bowl often, until creamy.
6. Add 1 egg at a time, beating well after each addition. Add vanilla; beat until well mixed. Add lemon zest and lemon juice until combined.
7. Stir together gluten-free flour blend and baking powder in small bowl.
8. Gradually add flour blend mixture alternately with milk to butter mixture, beating at low speed until well mixed.
9. Fold in the blueberries.
10. Pour batter into prepared pan. Bake for 50 to 60 minutes or until toothpick inserted in center comes out clean.
11. Cool 10 minutes; remove from pan.

12. Combine the powdered sugar and lemon juice in a small bowl and whisk until smooth.
13. Drizzle over the cake.
14. Serve and enjoy!

Gluten Free Coffee Cake

Ingredients:

2 tbsp. coconut oil
1 egg
1 tsp. vanilla extract
1/4 cup honey
1 1/2 cup almond flour
1 tsp. cinnamon
2 tsps. baking powder
1/2 cup coconut milk
1/2 tsp. sea salt
1/2 cup almond flour (for topping)
1 1/2 tbsp. coconut oil (for topping)
1 tbsp. honey (for topping)
2 tsps. cinnamon (for topping)

Directions:

1. Preheat oven to 350 degrees F.
2. Stir coconut oil, egg, vanilla and honey together in a bowl.
3. In a small bowl, combine almond flour, cinnamon, baking powder and sea salt.
4. Add dry ingredients to wet, along with coconut milk, and stir until smooth.
5. Pour into an 8×8 baking pan.
6. In a small bowl, mix the almond flour, coconut oil, honey and cinnamon for topping.
7. Spread the topping over the cake.
8. Bake for 20–25 minutes.

About the Author

Laura Sommers is **The Recipe Lady!**

She is the #1 Best Selling Author of over 80 recipe books.

She is a loving wife and mother who lives on a small farm in Baltimore County, Maryland and has a passion for all things domestic especially when it comes to saving money. She has a profitable eBay business and is a couponing addict. Follow her tips and tricks to learn how to make delicious meals on a budget, save money or to learn the latest life hack!

Visit her Amazon Author Page to see her latest books:

amazon.com/author/laurasommers

Visit the Recipe Lady's blog for even more great recipes and to learn which books are FREE for download each week:

http://the-recipe-lady.blogspot.com/

Follow the Recipe Lady on **Pinterest**:

http://pinterest.com/therecipelady1

Subscribe to The Recipe Lady blog through Amazon and have recipes and updates sent directly to your Kindle:

The Recipe Lady Blog through Amazon

Other books in This Series

- **Gluten Free Christmas Recipes**
- **Gluten Free Baking Recipes**
- **Gluten Free Cookie Recipes**
- **Gluten Free Cauliflower Recipes**
- **Gluten Free Cake Recipes**
- **Gluten Free Bread Recipes**

May all of your meals be a banquet
with good friends and good food.

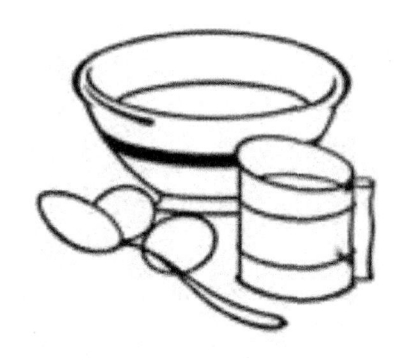

Printed in Great Britain
by Amazon